AUTOIMMUNE PALEO COOKBOOK

Mary Dixon

Copyright © 2023 by Dr. Mary Dixon

All rights reserved. No part of this publication may be reproduced, distributed, or transmitted in any form or by any means, including photocopying, recording, or other electronic or mechanical methods, without the prior written permission of the publisher, except in the case of brief quotation embodied in critical reviews and certain other non-commercial uses permitted by copyright law.

TABLE OF CONTENT

CHAPTER ONE

Auoimmune Diet and Benefits

Following an autoimmune diet, such as the Autoimmune Paleo (AIP) diet, can offer several benefits for those dealing with autoimmune conditions.

Here's a step-by-step guide on how to follow an autoimmune diet effectively to maximize its benefits:

1. Consult a Healthcare Professional: Before starting any diet, especially one as restrictive as AIP, consult with a healthcare professional or a registered dietitian who specializes in autoimmune diseases.

They can help you understand if the diet is appropriate for your specific condition and provide personalized guidance.

2. Educate Yourself: Learn about the AIP diet and its principles. Understand which foods are allowed and which are eliminated.

The AIP diet typically excludes grains, legumes, dairy, processed foods, sugar, nightshade vegetables, and certain spices.

3. Plan Your Meals: Create a meal plan that includes a variety of nutrient-dense foods that are allowed on the AIP diet.

Focus on consuming plenty of vegetables, fruits, lean meats, fish, healthy fats (such as avocado and olive oil), and bone broth.

4. Gradual Elimination: If you're transitioning from a standard diet, consider gradually eliminating the restricted foods over a week or two to make the adjustment more manageable.

5. Monitor Your Symptoms: Keep a journal to track your symptoms, energy levels, and overall well-being as you follow the AIP diet. This will help you gauge the diet's effectiveness and identify any trigger foods.

6. Stay Hydrated: Drink plenty of water to stay hydrated and support your body's detoxification processes.

7. Include AIP-Friendly Supplements: Depending on your specific needs and your healthcare provider's recommendations, consider including AIP-friendly supplements such as probiotics, omega-3 fatty acids, and vitamins/minerals to support your immune system and gut health.

8. Focus on Gut Health: Gut health is often linked to autoimmune conditions. Incorporate fermented foods like sauerkraut, kombucha, and kefir into your diet to promote a healthy gut microbiome.

9. Manage Stress: High-stress levels can exacerbate autoimmune symptoms. Practice stress-reduction techniques like meditation, yoga, or mindfulness to support your overall well-being.

10. Get Enough Sleep: Prioritize getting adequate sleep as it plays a crucial role in immune function and overall health.

11. Seek Support: Join online communities, support groups, or forums where individuals with autoimmune conditions share their experiences, recipes, and tips for following the AIP diet. This can provide motivation and help you navigate challenges.

12. Reintroduction Phase: After a period of strict AIP adherence (typically several weeks to months), work with your healthcare provider to gradually reintroduce eliminated foods one at a time. This process can help identify specific triggers for your autoimmune symptoms.

Remember that the AIP diet may not work the same way for everyone, and individual responses vary. Be patient and persistent in your efforts, and continue to work closely with your healthcare team to fine-tune your dietary approach.

The goal is to find a sustainable eating pattern that helps manage your autoimmune condition and supports your overall health and well-being.

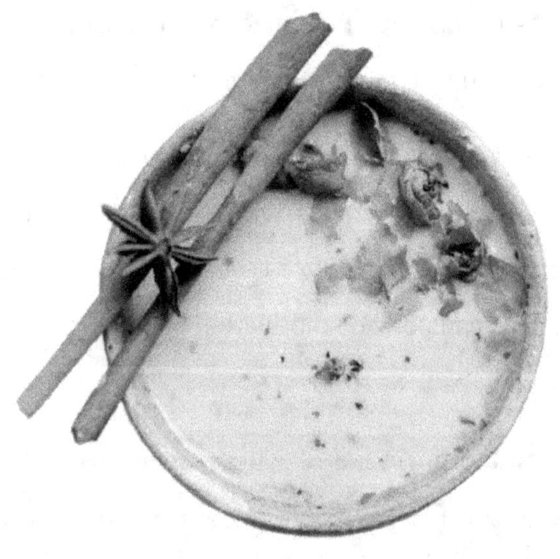

CHAPTER TWO

14-Day Autoimmune Diet Meal Plan

Creating a comprehensive 14-day autoimmune diet meal plan can be beneficial for individuals looking to follow the Autoimmune Paleo (AIP) diet.

Remember to consult with a healthcare professional or registered dietitian before starting any new diet, especially one as restrictive as AIP, to ensure it is suitable for your specific needs.

Day 1:

- Breakfast: Scrambled eggs with spinach and avocado.
- Lunch: Grilled chicken salad with mixed greens, carrots, and a lemon-turmeric dressing.
- Dinner: Baked salmon with roasted asparagus and sweet potato.

Day 2:

- Breakfast: AIP-friendly smoothie with coconut milk, berries, and collagen powder.

- Lunch: Zucchini noodles with homemade pesto (made without nuts) and cherry tomatoes.
- Dinner: Beef stew with carrots, celery, and bone broth.

Day 3:

- Breakfast: Sautéed kale with garlic, bacon, and poached eggs.
- Lunch: Turkey and avocado lettuce wraps with a side of sliced cucumber.
- Dinner: Baked cod with a lemon-herb sauce, served with steamed broccoli and cauliflower.

Day 4:

- Breakfast: AIP-friendly pumpkin pancakes with coconut yogurt and fresh berries.
- Lunch: Tuna salad made with canned tuna, avocado, red onion, and a lemon-olive oil dressing.
- Dinner: Grilled lamb chops with roasted Brussels sprouts and mashed cauliflower.

Day 5:

- Breakfast: Sweet potato hash with ground turkey, spinach, and turmeric.

- Lunch: Chicken and vegetable soup made with bone broth.

- Dinner: Baked chicken thighs with roasted butternut squash and sautéed kale.

Day 6:

- Breakfast: AIP-friendly banana muffins with coconut butter.

- Lunch: Shredded pork lettuce wraps with homemade slaw.

- Dinner: Baked halibut with a garlic and parsley sauce, served with sautéed spinach.

Day 7:

- Breakfast: AIP-friendly green smoothie with kale, cucumber, and pineapple.

- Lunch: Roast beef salad with mixed greens, radishes, and a balsamic vinaigrette.

- Dinner: Turkey meatballs with AIP-friendly marinara sauce over spaghetti squash.

Day 8:

- Breakfast: Scrambled eggs with sautéed mushrooms and a side of sliced kiwi.

- Lunch: Salmon and avocado salad with mixed greens and a lemon-turmeric dressing.
- Dinner: Grilled pork chops with mashed sweet potatoes and steamed broccoli.

Day 9:

- Breakfast: AIP-friendly coconut yogurt with sliced banana and a sprinkle of cinnamon.
- Lunch: Turkey and vegetable stir-fry with coconut aminos.
- Dinner: Baked chicken drumsticks with roasted carrots and parsnips.

Day 10:

- Breakfast: AIP-friendly blueberry muffins with coconut butter.
- Lunch: Tuna and avocado salad with diced cucumber and lemon-olive oil dressing.
- Dinner: Beef and vegetable kabobs with grilled zucchini and red bell peppers.

Day 11:

- Breakfast: Scrambled eggs with sautéed kale and a side of mixed berries.

- Lunch: Chicken soup with carrots, celery, and cauliflower rice.
- Dinner: Baked cod with a dill and lemon sauce, served with roasted asparagus.

Day 12:

- Breakfast: AIP-friendly smoothie with coconut milk, mango, and collagen powder.
- Lunch: Turkey lettuce wraps with homemade guacamole and sliced radishes.
- Dinner: Grilled lamb burgers with sweet potato fries and a side of sautéed spinach.

Day 13:

- Breakfast: Sweet potato and bacon hash with poached eggs.
- Lunch: Chicken and vegetable stir-fry with broccoli, carrots, and coconut aminos.
- Dinner: Baked chicken thighs with roasted Brussels sprouts and mashed cauliflower.

Day 14:

- Breakfast: AIP-friendly pumpkin pancakes with coconut yogurt and fresh berries.

- Lunch: Shredded pork and coleslaw lettuce wraps with a side of sliced cucumber.
- Dinner: Grilled halibut with a garlic and parsley sauce, served with sautéed kale.

Remember to stay hydrated throughout the day, and feel free to adjust portion sizes and ingredients to meet your dietary needs and preferences. It's essential to consult with a healthcare professional or registered dietitian for personalized guidance on following the AIP diet effectively.

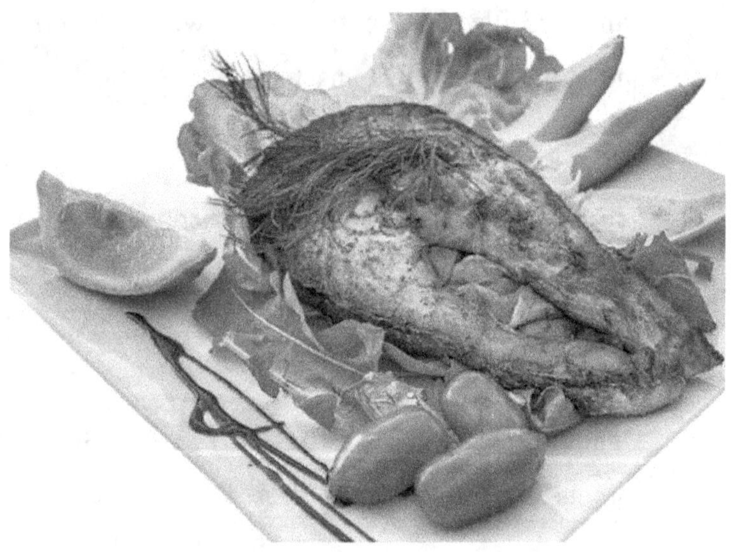

CHAPTER THREE

Autoimmune Diet Breakfast Recipes

1. Sweet Potato and Turkey Hash

Start your day with a savory and satisfying hash that's AIP-friendly.

Ingredients:

- 1 medium sweet potato, peeled and diced
- 1/2 lb ground turkey
- 1/2 onion, chopped
- 1 garlic clove, minced
- 1 tsp dried thyme
- Salt and pepper to taste
- Avocado oil for cooking

Instructions:

1. Heat avocado oil in a skillet over medium heat.

2. Add onions and garlic; sauté until fragrant.

3. Add ground turkey and cook until browned.

4. Add sweet potatoes and thyme; cook until potatoes are tender.

5. Season with salt and pepper.

6. Serve hot.

Cooking Time: Approximately 20 minutes.

2. AIP Breakfast Bowl

This breakfast bowl combines nutritious ingredients for a hearty start to your day.

Ingredients:

- 1/2 cup cooked ground turkey
- 1/2 cup cooked spinach
- 1/2 avocado, sliced
- 1/2 cup mashed sweet potatoes
- Fresh herbs for garnish (e.g., parsley or cilantro)
- Olive oil for drizzling

Instructions:

1. Place cooked ground turkey at the bottom of a bowl.

2. Top with cooked spinach and mashed sweet potatoes.

3. Add avocado slices.

4. Garnish with fresh herbs and a drizzle of olive oil.

Cooking Time: Varies depending on pre-cooked ingredients.

3. AIP-Friendly Smoothie Bowl

This vibrant smoothie bowl is packed with nutrient-rich ingredients to kickstart your day.

Ingredients:

- 1 ripe banana
- 1/2 cup frozen mixed berries
- 1/2 cup unsweetened coconut yogurt (AIP-compliant)
- 1 tbsp collagen powder
- 1/2 cup coconut milk
- Fresh berries and shredded coconut for topping

Instructions:

1. Blend banana, frozen berries, coconut yogurt, collagen powder, and coconut milk until smooth.

2. Pour into a bowl and top with fresh berries and shredded coconut.

Cooking Time: 5 minutes (preparation time).

4. Apple Cinnamon Porridge

Enjoy a comforting bowl of hot porridge without grains or dairy.

Ingredients:

- 1 medium apple, peeled and grated
- 2 tbsp coconut flour
- 1/2 tsp cinnamon
- 1/2 cup coconut milk
- 1 tbsp honey (optional)
- Sliced almonds for garnish (optional)

Instructions:

1. In a saucepan, combine grated apple, coconut flour, cinnamon, and coconut milk.

2. Cook over low heat, stirring until the mixture thickens.

3. Sweeten with honey if desired.

4. Serve hot, garnished with sliced almonds.

Cooking Time: Approximately 10 minutes.

5. Turkey and Vegetable Scramble

This protein-packed scramble is a savory and satisfying way to start your day.

Ingredients:

- 2 large eggs (if tolerated)
- 1/2 cup cooked ground turkey
- 1/2 cup sautéed spinach
- 1/4 cup diced zucchini
- Salt and pepper to taste
- Avocado oil for cooking

Instructions:

1. Heat avocado oil in a skillet over medium heat.

2. Add diced zucchini and sauté until tender.

3. Add cooked ground turkey and sautéed spinach.

4. Beat the eggs (if tolerated) and pour them into the skillet.

5. Cook until the eggs are set, stirring occasionally.

6. Season with salt and pepper.

7. Serve hot.

Cooking Time: Approximately 10 minutes.

6. Coconut and Berry Parfait

Indulge in a dairy-free parfait that's both delicious and autoimmune-friendly.

Ingredients:

- 1/2 cup unsweetened coconut yogurt (AIP-compliant)
- 1/2 cup mixed berries (e.g., blueberries, strawberries)

- 1 tbsp shredded coconut
- 1 tsp honey (optional)

Instructions:

1. In a glass or bowl, layer coconut yogurt and mixed berries.

2. Top with shredded coconut.

3. Drizzle with honey if desired.

4. Serve chilled.

Cooking Time: Varies depending on preparation.

7. Plantain Pancakes

These fluffy plantain pancakes are a delightful twist on traditional pancakes.

Ingredients:

- 2 ripe plantains
- 2 large eggs (if tolerated)
- 1/2 tsp cinnamon
- 1/4 tsp baking soda
- Avocado oil for cooking

Instructions:

1. Peel and slice the plantains, then blend them with eggs (if tolerated), cinnamon, and baking soda until smooth.

2. Heat avocado oil in a skillet over medium heat.

3. Pour small portions of the batter onto the skillet to make pancakes.

4. Cook until golden brown on both sides.

5. Serve hot.

Cooking Time: Approximately 15 minutes.

8. Chicken and Vegetable Breakfast Soup

Start your day with a nourishing bowl of chicken and vegetable soup.

Ingredients:

- 1 cup homemade chicken broth
- 1/2 cup shredded chicken breast
- 1/2 cup diced carrots
- 1/2 cup diced celery
- Fresh herbs for garnish (e.g., parsley or dill)

Instructions:

1. In a saucepan, combine chicken broth, shredded chicken, diced carrots, and celery.

2. Simmer until the vegetables are tender.

3. Garnish with fresh herbs.

4. Serve hot.

Cooking Time: Approximately 20 minutes.

9. Mixed Berry and Spinach Salad

This refreshing salad is a light and nutritious option for breakfast.

Ingredients:

- 2 cups fresh mixed berries (e.g., raspberries, blackberries, blueberries)
- 1 cup fresh spinach leaves
- 1 tbsp balsamic vinegar (check ingredients for compliance)
- 1 tsp olive oil

Instructions:

1. Toss mixed berries and spinach in a bowl.

2. Drizzle with balsamic vinegar and olive oil.

3. Gently toss to combine.

4. Serve chilled.

Cooking Time: Varies depending on preparation.

10. Cucumber and Avocado Boat

A quick and refreshing breakfast that's perfect for hot mornings.

Ingredients:

- 1 cucumber, halved and seeds scooped out
- 1/2 avocado, diced
- Sliced radishes for garnish
- Fresh herbs (e.g., mint or cilantro)
- Olive oil and lemon juice for drizzling

Instructions:

1. Scoop out the seeds from the cucumber halves to create boats.

2. Fill each cucumber boat with diced avocado.

3. Garnish with sliced radishes and fresh herbs.

4. Drizzle with olive oil and lemon juice.

5. Serve chilled.

Cooking Time: Varies depending on preparation.

Autoimmune Diet Lunch Recipes

1. AIP Chicken and Vegetable Stir-Fry

This colorful stir-fry is packed with nutrient-rich vegetables and protein for a satisfying autoimmune diet lunch.

Ingredients:

- 1 boneless, skinless chicken breast, thinly sliced
- 2 cups broccoli florets
- 1 cup sliced carrots
- 1 cup sliced bell peppers
- 2 cloves garlic, minced
- 2 tbsp coconut aminos
- 1 tbsp coconut oil
- Salt and pepper to taste

Instructions:

1. Heat coconut oil in a skillet over medium-high heat.

2. Add sliced chicken and cook until browned.

3. Add minced garlic and cook for another minute.

4. Add broccoli, carrots, and bell peppers. Stir-fry until vegetables are tender.

5. Drizzle with coconut aminos and season with salt and pepper.

6. Serve hot.

Cooking Time: Approximately 20 minutes.

2. AIP Salmon Salad

Enjoy a light and refreshing salad with baked salmon and a citrusy dressing.

Ingredients:

- 1 salmon fillet
- 4 cups mixed greens (AIP-compliant)
- 1/2 cucumber, thinly sliced
- 1/4 red onion, thinly sliced
- Juice of 1 lemon
- 2 tbsp olive oil
- Fresh dill for garnish
- Salt and pepper to taste

Instructions:

1. Preheat the oven to 375°F (190°C).

2. Season the salmon fillet with salt and pepper.

3. Bake for 15-20 minutes until the salmon flakes easily.

4. In a bowl, combine mixed greens, cucumber, and red onion.

5. Whisk together lemon juice and olive oil to make the dressing.

6. Flake the baked salmon and add it to the salad.

7. Drizzle with the dressing and garnish with fresh dill.

8. Serve chilled.

Cooking Time: Approximately 20 minutes.

3. AIP Turkey and Avocado Wrap

This AIP-friendly wrap is a convenient and satisfying option for lunch.

Ingredients:

- 4 large lettuce leaves (e.g., iceberg or butter lettuce)
- 1/2 lb ground turkey
- 1/2 avocado, sliced
- 1/2 cup shredded carrots
- Olive oil for cooking
- Salt and pepper to taste

Instructions:

1. Heat olive oil in a skillet over medium heat.

2. Add ground turkey and cook until browned.

3. Season with salt and pepper.

4. Assemble the wraps by placing cooked turkey, avocado slices, and shredded carrots on lettuce leaves.

5. Roll up the leaves and secure with toothpicks if needed.

6. Serve immediately.

Cooking Time: Approximately 15 minutes.

4. AIP Beef and Vegetable Soup

Warm up with a comforting bowl of AIP-friendly beef and vegetable soup.

Ingredients:

- 1/2 lb ground beef
- 4 cups bone broth (AIP-compliant)
- 2 cups diced sweet potatoes
- 1 cup sliced celery
- 1 cup sliced carrots
- 1 cup diced zucchini
- 1 tsp dried thyme
- Salt and pepper to taste

- Fresh parsley for garnish

Instructions:

1. In a soup pot, brown the ground beef over medium heat.

2. Add sweet potatoes, celery, carrots, and zucchini.

3. Pour in the bone broth and add dried thyme.

4. Season with salt and pepper.

5. Simmer until the vegetables are tender.

6. Garnish with fresh parsley.

7. Serve hot.

Cooking Time: Approximately 30 minutes.

5. AIP Tuna Salad

This AIP-friendly tuna salad is a quick and satisfying lunch option.

Ingredients:

- 2 cans of AIP-compliant canned tuna, drained
- 1/2 avocado, mashed
- 1/4 red onion, finely chopped
- 1/4 cucumber, finely chopped

- 2 tbsp olive oil

- Juice of 1 lemon

- Fresh dill for garnish

- Salt and pepper to taste

Instructions:

1. In a bowl, combine drained tuna, mashed avocado, chopped red onion, and chopped cucumber.

2. Drizzle with olive oil and lemon juice.

3. Season with salt and pepper.

4. Garnish with fresh dill.

5. Serve chilled.

Cooking Time: No cooking required.

6. AIP Turkey and Sweet Potato Hash

This hash is a hearty and flavorful option for an AIP-friendly lunch.

Ingredients:

- 1/2 lb ground turkey

- 1 medium sweet potato, peeled and diced

- 1/2 onion, chopped

- 1/2 cup sliced mushrooms

- 2 cloves garlic, minced

- 2 tbsp coconut oil

- Salt and pepper to taste

Instructions:

1. Heat coconut oil in a skillet over medium heat.

2. Add chopped onion and minced garlic; sauté until fragrant.

3. Add ground turkey and cook until browned.

4. Add diced sweet potato and sliced mushrooms.

5. Cook until sweet potatoes are tender.

6. Season with salt and pepper.

7. Serve hot.

Cooking Time: Approximately 25 minutes.

7. AIP Avocado and Shrimp Salad

Enjoy a light and protein-packed shrimp salad with creamy avocado.

Ingredients:

- 1/2 lb cooked and peeled shrimp

- 2 ripe avocados, diced

- 1 cup cherry tomatoes, halved

- Fresh basil leaves for garnish

- Olive oil and balsamic vinegar (AIP-compliant) for drizzling

- Salt and pepper to taste

Instructions:

1. In a bowl, combine cooked shrimp, diced avocado, and halved cherry tomatoes.

2. Drizzle with olive oil and balsamic vinegar.

3. Season with salt and pepper.

4. Garnish with fresh basil leaves.

5. Serve chilled.

Cooking Time: Varies depending on pre-cooked shrimp.

8. AIP Chicken and Kale Salad

This salad is a nutritious and satisfying choice for an AIP-friendly lunch.

Ingredients:

- 1 boneless, skinless chicken breast, grilled and sliced
- 2 cups chopped kale
- 1/2 cup shredded carrots
- 1/4 cup sliced almonds
- Juice of 1 lemon
- 2 tbsp olive oil
- Salt and pepper to taste

Instructions:

1. In a bowl, massage chopped kale with lemon juice and olive oil until slightly softened.

2. Add grilled chicken, shredded carrots, and sliced almonds.

3. Season with salt and pepper.

4. Toss to combine.

5. Serve chilled.

Cooking Time: Approximately 15 minutes (grilling time not included).

9. AIP Roast Beef and Radish Salad

This salad features tender roast beef and crisp radishes for a flavorful lunch.

Ingredients:

- 1 cup thinly sliced roast beef
- 1 cup sliced radishes
- 1/4 red onion, thinly sliced
- Fresh parsley for garnish
- Olive oil and lemon juice for drizzling
- Salt and pepper to taste

Instructions:

1. In a bowl, combine thinly sliced roast beef, sliced radishes, and thinly sliced red onion.

2. Drizzle with olive oil and lemon juice.

3. Season with salt and pepper.

4. Garnish with fresh parsley.

5. Serve chilled.

Cooking Time: Varies depending on pre-cooked roast beef.

10. AIP Cauliflower Rice and Ground Pork Stir-Fry

This cauliflower rice stir-fry is a low-carb and flavorful lunch option.

Ingredients:

- 1/2 lb ground pork
- 1 small head of cauliflower, riced
- 1/2 cup diced bell peppers
- 1/2 cup sliced green onions
- 2 cloves garlic, minced
- 2 tbsp coconut aminos
- 1 tbsp coconut oil
- Salt and pepper to taste

Instructions:

1. Heat coconut oil in a skillet over medium heat.

2. Add minced garlic and diced bell peppers; sauté until tender.

3. Add ground pork and cook until browned.

4. Stir in cauliflower rice and sliced green onions.

5. Drizzle with coconut aminos.

6. Season with salt and pepper.

7. Stir-fry until cauliflower rice is heated through.

8. Serve hot.

Cooking Time: Approximately 20 minutes.

These AIP-friendly lunch recipes offer variety and flavor while adhering to autoimmune protocol guidelines. Adjust the recipes to suit your preferences.

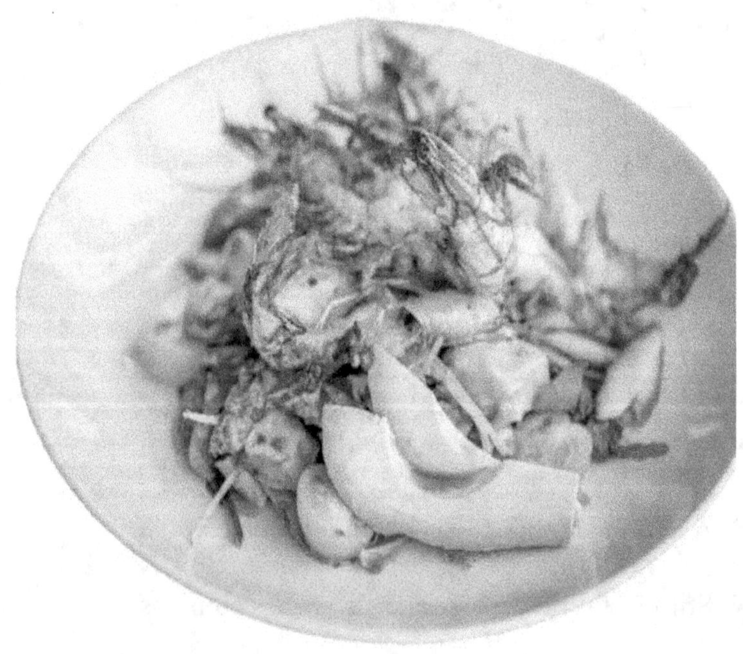

CHAPTER FOUR

Autoimmune Diet Dinner Recipes

1. AIP Lemon Herb Baked Chicken

This flavorful and aromatic baked chicken is a simple yet satisfying dinner option.

Ingredients:

- 4 boneless, skinless chicken thighs
- Zest and juice of 1 lemon
- 2 cloves garlic, minced
- 1 tsp dried thyme
- 1 tsp dried rosemary
- Salt and pepper to taste
- Olive oil for drizzling

Instructions:

1. Preheat the oven to 375°F (190°C).

2. In a bowl, mix lemon zest, lemon juice, minced garlic, dried thyme, dried rosemary, salt, and pepper.

3. Place chicken thighs in a baking dish and pour the lemon herb mixture over them.

4. Drizzle with olive oil.

5. Bake for approximately 25-30 minutes or until the chicken is cooked through and golden brown.

6. Serve hot.

Cooking Time: Approximately 30 minutes.

2. AIP Baked Salmon with Cilantro-Lime Sauce

Enjoy a delicious and nutritious salmon dish with a zesty cilantro-lime sauce.

Ingredients:

- 4 salmon fillets
- Zest and juice of 1 lime
- 1/4 cup fresh cilantro, chopped
- 2 cloves garlic, minced
- 2 tbsp olive oil
- Salt and pepper to taste

Instructions:

1. Preheat the oven to 375°F (190°C).

2. Season salmon fillets with salt and pepper and place them in a baking dish.

3. In a bowl, combine lime zest, lime juice, chopped cilantro, minced garlic, and olive oil.

4. Pour the cilantro-lime mixture over the salmon.

5. Bake for approximately 15-20 minutes or until the salmon flakes easily.

6. Serve hot.

Cooking Time: Approximately 20 minutes.

3. AIP Turkey and Sweet Potato Skillet

This one-pan turkey and sweet potato skillet is a quick and satisfying dinner option.

Ingredients:

- 1 lb ground turkey
- 2 medium sweet potatoes, peeled and diced
- 1/2 onion, chopped
- 1 tsp dried sage
- 1 tsp dried thyme
- Salt and pepper to taste
- Avocado oil for cooking

Instructions:

1. Heat avocado oil in a large skillet over medium-high heat.

2. Add chopped onion and cook until translucent.

3. Add ground turkey and cook until browned.

4. Add diced sweet potatoes, dried sage, dried thyme, salt, and pepper.

5. Cook until sweet potatoes are tender and turkey is cooked through.

6. Serve hot.

Cooking Time: Approximately 20 minutes.

4. AIP Zucchini Noodles with AIP Pesto

Enjoy a satisfying and pesto-infused zucchini noodle dish that's both flavorful and autoimmune-friendly.

Ingredients:

- 2 large zucchinis, spiralized into noodles
- 1/2 cup fresh basil leaves
- 1/4 cup chopped parsley
- 1/4 cup chopped cilantro

- 2 cloves garlic, minced

- 1/4 cup olive oil

- 1/4 cup coconut cream

- Salt and pepper to taste

- Sliced cherry tomatoes for garnish (optional)

Instructions:

1. In a blender or food processor, combine fresh basil, chopped parsley, chopped cilantro, minced garlic, olive oil, and coconut cream.

2. Blend until a smooth pesto sauce forms.

3. In a large skillet, sauté zucchini noodles until tender.

4. Toss the cooked zucchini noodles with the pesto sauce.

5. Season with salt and pepper.

6. Garnish with sliced cherry tomatoes if desired.

7. Serve hot.

Cooking Time: Approximately 15 minutes.

5. AIP Slow Cooker Beef Stew

This hearty and comforting beef stew is prepared in a slow cooker for convenience.

Ingredients:

- 1.5 lbs beef stew meat, cubed
- 2 cups diced carrots
- 2 cups diced celery
- 2 cups diced sweet potatoes
- 1 onion, chopped
- 4 cups bone broth (AIP-compliant)
- 2 tsp dried thyme
- 2 tsp dried rosemary
- Salt and pepper to taste

Instructions:

1. Place beef stew meat, diced carrots, diced celery, diced sweet potatoes, and chopped onion in a slow cooker.

2. Pour bone broth over the ingredients.

3. Add dried thyme, dried rosemary, salt, and pepper.

4. Stir to combine.

5. Cook on low for 6-8 hours or until beef and vegetables are tender.

6. Serve hot.

Cooking Time: Approximately 6-8 hours (slow cooker).

6. AIP Lemon-Garlic Shrimp and Asparagus

This zesty and vibrant shrimp and asparagus dish is a quick and flavorful dinner option.

Ingredients:

- 1 lb large shrimp, peeled and deveined
- 1 bunch asparagus, trimmed and cut into pieces
- Zest and juice of 1 lemon
- 3 cloves garlic, minced
- 2 tbsp olive oil
- Salt and pepper to taste

Instructions:

1. In a bowl, combine shrimp, asparagus pieces, lemon zest, lemon juice, minced garlic, olive oil, salt, and pepper.

2. Toss to coat the shrimp and asparagus.

3. Heat a large skillet over medium-high heat.

4. Add the shrimp and asparagus mixture to the skillet.

5. Sauté for approximately 5-7 minutes or until shrimp are pink and cooked through.

6. Serve hot.

Cooking Time: Approximately 10 minutes.

7. AIP Grilled Chicken with Avocado Salsa

Enjoy a light and refreshing grilled chicken dish with a flavorful avocado salsa.

Ingredients:

- 4 boneless, skinless chicken breasts
- 2 ripe avocados, diced
- 1/2 red onion, finely chopped
- 1/4 cup chopped fresh cilantro
- Juice of 2 limes
- Salt and pepper to taste

Instructions:

1. Preheat the grill to medium-high heat.

2. Season chicken breasts with salt and pepper.

3. Grill chicken for approximately 6-8 minutes per side or until cooked through.

4. In a bowl, combine diced avocado, chopped red onion, chopped cilantro, and lime juice to make the salsa.

5. Season the salsa with salt and pepper.

6. Serve grilled chicken topped with avocado salsa.

7. Serve hot.

Cooking Time: Approximately 15-20 minutes.

8. AIP Baked Cod with Garlic and Herbs

This baked cod with garlic and herbs is a flavorful and light dinner option.

Ingredients:

- 4 cod fillets
- 2 cloves garlic, minced
- 2 tbsp chopped fresh parsley
- 2 tbsp chopped fresh chives
- 2 tbsp olive oil
- Zest and juice of 1 lemo
- Salt and pepper to taste

Instructions:

1. Preheat the oven to 375°F (190°C).

2. Place cod fillets in a baking dish.

3. In a bowl, combine minced garlic, chopped fresh parsley, chopped fresh chives, olive oil, lemon zest, lemon juice, salt, and pepper.

4. Pour the herb and garlic mixture over the cod fillets.

5. Bake for approximately 15-20 minutes or until the cod flakes easily.

6. Serve hot.

Cooking Time: Approximately 20 minutes.

9. AIP Turkey Meatballs with AIP Marinara Sauce

These AIP-friendly turkey meatballs are served with a flavorful marinara sauce.

Ingredients:

- 1 lb ground turkey
- 1/4 cup chopped fresh basil

- 1/4 cup chopped fresh parsley

- 2 cloves garlic, minced

- 1/4 cup finely chopped onion

- Salt and pepper to taste

- 2 cups AIP-compliant marinara sauce

Instructions:

1. Preheat the oven to 375°F (190°C).

2. In a bowl, combine ground turkey, chopped fresh basil, chopped fresh parsley, minced garlic, chopped onion, salt, and pepper.

3. Form the mixture into meatballs and place them in a baking dish.

4. Pour AIP-compliant marinara sauce over the meatballs.

5. Bake for approximately 25-30 minutes or until the meatballs are cooked through.

6. Serve hot.

Cooking Time: Approximately 30 minutes.

10. AIP Slow Cooker Pork Roast with Vegetables

This slow cooker pork roast with vegetables is a flavorful and convenient dinner option.

Ingredients:

- 2 lbs boneless pork roast
- 4 cups diced sweet potatoes
- 2 cups diced carrots
- 1 onion, chopped
- 2 cloves garlic, minced
- 2 tsp dried thyme
- 2 tsp dried rosemary
- Salt and pepper to taste
- 1 cup bone broth (AIP-compliant)

Instructions:

1. Place boneless pork roast in a slow cooker.

2. Add diced sweet potatoes, diced carrots, chopped onion, minced garlic, dried thyme, dried rosemary, salt, and pepper.

3. Pour bone broth over the ingredients.

4. Cook on low for 6-8 hours or until the pork is tender and vegetables are cooked through.

5. Serve hot.

Cooking Time: Approximately 6-8 hours (slow cooker).

Autoimmune Diet Snack Recipes

1. AIP Guacamole with Veggie Sticks

This guacamole paired with colorful vegetable sticks makes for a satisfying and healthy autoimmune diet snack.

Ingredients:

- 2 ripe avocados
- Juice of 1 lime
- 2 cloves garlic, minced
- 2 tbsp chopped fresh cilantro
- Salt and pepper to taste
- Assorted vegetable sticks (carrots, celery, cucumber

Instructions:

1. In a bowl, mash the ripe avocados.

2. Add lime juice, minced garlic, chopped fresh cilantro, salt, and pepper.

3. Mix until well combined.

4. Serve with vegetable sticks for dipping.

Preparation Time: Approximately 10 minutes.

2. AIP Roasted Plantain Chips

These crispy roasted plantain chips are a delicious alternative to regular potato chips.

Ingredients:

- 2 ripe plantains
- 2 tbsp avocado oil
- Salt to taste

Instructions:

1. Preheat the oven to 350°F (175°C).

2. Peel the ripe plantains and slice them thinly.

3. In a bowl, toss the plantain slices with avocado oil and salt.

4. Spread the plantain slices in a single layer on a baking sheet.

5. Bake for approximately 20-25 minutes, flipping them halfway through, until they are crisp and golden.

6. Let them cool before enjoying.

Preparation Time: Approximately 30 minutes.

3. AIP Turkey and Cranberry Lettuce Wraps

These refreshing lettuce wraps combine turkey and cranberry for a tasty autoimmune diet snack.

Ingredients:

- 1/2 lb ground turkey
- 1/4 cup AIP-friendly cranberry sauce
- 8 large lettuce leaves (e.g., iceberg or butter lettuce)
- Sliced green onions for garnish

Instructions:

1. In a skillet, cook ground turkey until browned.

2. Stir in AIP-friendly cranberry sauce and cook for an additional minute.

3. Spoon the turkey mixture into lettuce leaves.

4. Garnish with sliced green onions.

5. Serve immediately.

Preparation Time: Approximately 15 minutes.

4. AIP Coconut-Covered Dates

These sweet and satisfying coconut-covered dates are a simple and enjoyable autoimmune diet snack.

Ingredients:

- 10 Medjool dates, pitted
- 1/4 cup shredded coconut (AIP-compliant)

Instructions:

1. Gently open the pitted dates.

2. Stuff each date with shredded coconut.

3. Press the coconut onto the dates.

4. Serve immediately or refrigerate for a firmer texture.

Preparation Time: Approximately 10 minutes.

5. AIP Cucumber and Smoked Salmon Bites

These cucumber and smoked salmon bites are a refreshing and protein-rich snack option.

Ingredients:

- 1 cucumber, sliced into rounds
- Smoked salmon slices
- Fresh dill for garnish

Instructions:

1. Place a slice of smoked salmon on each cucumber round.

2. Garnish with fresh dill.

3. Serve chilled.

Preparation Time: Approximately 10 minutes.

6. AIP Carrot and Ginger Soup

This chilled carrot and ginger soup is a nutritious and refreshing autoimmune diet snack.

Ingredients:

- 2 cups cooked and mashed carrots
- 1 cup coconut milk (AIP-compliant)

- 1 tsp grated fresh ginger
- Salt and pepper to taste
- Fresh chives for garnish

Instructions:

1. In a blender, combine cooked and mashed carrots, coconut milk, grated fresh ginger, salt, and pepper.

2. Blend until smooth.

3. Refrigerate until chilled.

4. Garnish with fresh chives.

5. Serve cold.

Preparation Time: Approximately 15 minutes.

7. AIP Blueberry and Banana Smoothie

This AIP-friendly blueberry and banana smoothie is a quick and nutritious snack.

Ingredients:

- 1 ripe banana
- 1/2 cup frozen blueberries
- 1/2 cup coconut milk (AIP-compliant)

- 1/2 cup water

- 1 tbsp honey (optional)

Instructions:

1. Blend banana, frozen blueberries, coconut milk, and water until smooth.

2. Sweeten with honey if desired.

3. Pour into a glass and serve chilled.

Preparation Time: Approximately 5 minutes.

8. AIP Beef Jerky

This homemade beef jerky is a protein-packed and savory autoimmune diet snack.

Ingredients:

- 1 lb lean beef (e.g., top round or sirloin)

- 1/4 cup coconut aminos

- 1 tsp garlic powder

- 1 tsp onion powder

- 1 tsp smoked paprika

- Salt and pepper to taste

Instructions:

1. Slice the lean beef into thin strips.

2. In a bowl, combine coconut aminos, garlic powder, onion powder, smoked paprika, salt, and pepper.

3. Marinate the beef strips in the mixture for at least 2 hours or overnight in the refrigerator.

4. Preheat your oven to 175°F (80°C).

5. Place the marinated beef strips on a baking rack.

6. Bake for 3-4 hours or until the beef is dried and chewy.

7. Let it cool before enjoying.

Preparation Time: Approximately 4-6 hours (including marinating time).

9. AIP Baked Kale Chips

These crispy baked kale chips are a nutritious and crunchy autoimmune diet snack.

Ingredients:

- 1 bunch of kale, washed and dried
- 1 tbsp olive oil

- Salt and pepper to taste

Instructions:

1. Preheat the oven to 275°F (135°C).

2. Remove the stems from the kale leaves and tear them into bite-sized pieces.

3. In a bowl, toss kale pieces with olive oil, salt, and pepper.

4. Spread the kale pieces in a single layer on a baking sheet.

5. Bake for approximately 20-25 minutes or until the kale chips are crisp.

6. Let them cool before enjoying.

Preparation Time: Approximately 30 minutes.

10. AIP Berry Parfait

This berry parfait combines AIP-friendly ingredients for a sweet and satisfying snack.

Ingredients:

- 1 cup mixed berries (e.g., blueberries, raspberries)
- 1/2 cup coconut yogurt (AIP-compliant)
- 1/4 cup toasted coconut flakes (AIP-compliant)

-    1 tsp honey (optional)

Instructions:

1. In a glass, layer mixed berries and coconut yogurt.

2. Repeat the layers.

3. Top with toasted coconut flakes.

4. Sweeten with honey if desired.

5. Serve chilled.

Preparation Time: Approximately 10 minutes.

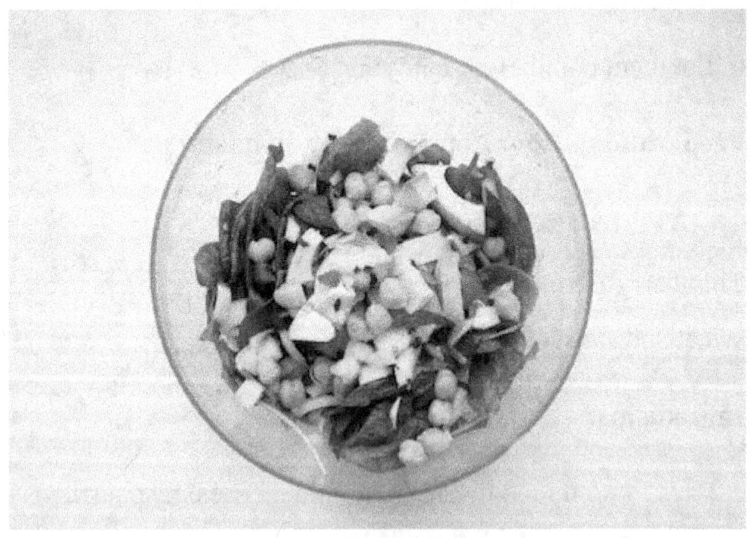

CONCLUSION

In conclusion, the autoimmune diet, often referred to as the Autoimmune Protocol (AIP), is a powerful dietary approach designed to alleviate symptoms and manage autoimmune diseases. It focuses on removing potential triggers and inflammatory foods while emphasizing nutrient-dense, healing foods. Here's a recap of some key takeaways from the autoimmune diet:

1. Elimination of Trigger Foods: One of the fundamental principles of the autoimmune diet is the elimination of foods that can trigger inflammation and worsen autoimmune symptoms. Common culprits include grains, legumes, dairy, processed sugars, and nightshades.

2. Nutrient-Dense Whole Foods: The diet places a strong emphasis on nutrient-dense whole foods such as lean proteins, fish rich in omega-3 fatty acids, a variety of colorful vegetables, and fruits. These foods provide essential vitamins, minerals, and antioxidants that support the immune system and promote overall health.

3. Gut Health: AIP recognizes the critical role of gut health in autoimmune conditions. It encourages the consumption of foods that support gut healing, like bone broth and fermented foods, to restore the balance of beneficial gut bacteria.

4. Anti-Inflammatory Herbs and Spices: Many herbs and spices with anti-inflammatory properties are staples in the autoimmune diet. Turmeric, ginger, and garlic, for example, are used to flavor dishes while providing potential therapeutic benefits.

5. Personalization: While AIP provides a general framework, it is highly adaptable and should be personalized to meet individual needs. Some people may need to reintroduce certain foods over time, while others may need stricter adherence to the protocol.

6. Consultation with Professionals: Before embarking on the autoimmune diet, it is essential to consult with healthcare professionals, including a registered dietitian or functional medicine practitioner. They can help tailor the diet to specific autoimmune conditions and ensure balanced nutrition.

7. Lifestyle Factors: While diet is a critical component, other lifestyle factors like stress management, sleep quality, and regular physical activity play a crucial role in managing autoimmune diseases. A holistic approach that addresses all aspects of well-being is often the most effective.

In summary, the autoimmune diet is not a one-size-fits-all solution, but rather a valuable tool for those seeking relief from autoimmune symptoms.

By eliminating trigger foods, embracing nutrient-dense options, and addressing gut health, individuals can empower themselves to take control of their autoimmune conditions and improve their overall quality of life.

However, it's essential to approach this dietary approach with guidance from healthcare professionals and to remember that results may vary from person to person. The autoimmune diet represents an opportunity to harness the healing power of food and make informed choices that support long-term health and well-being.

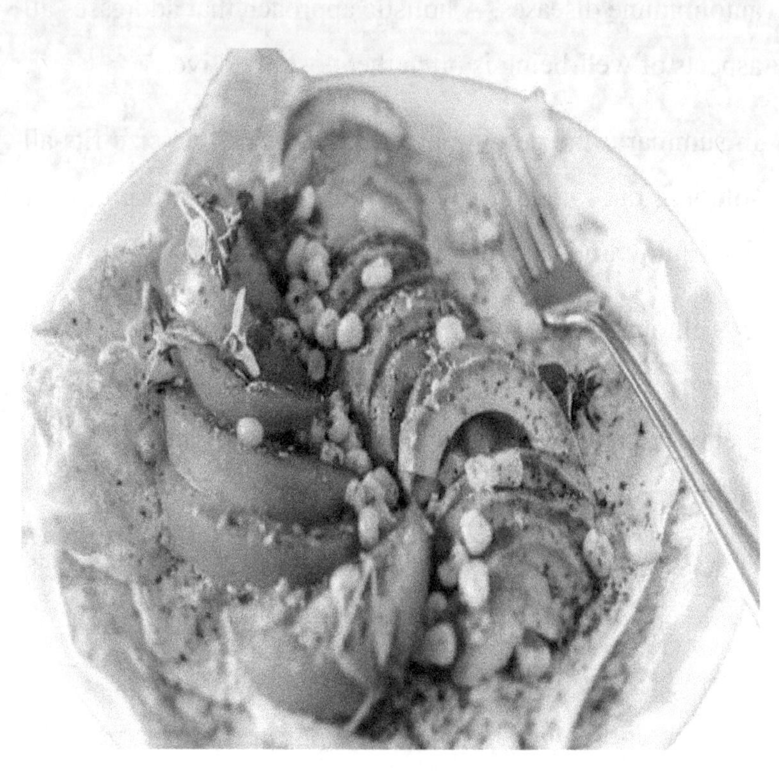

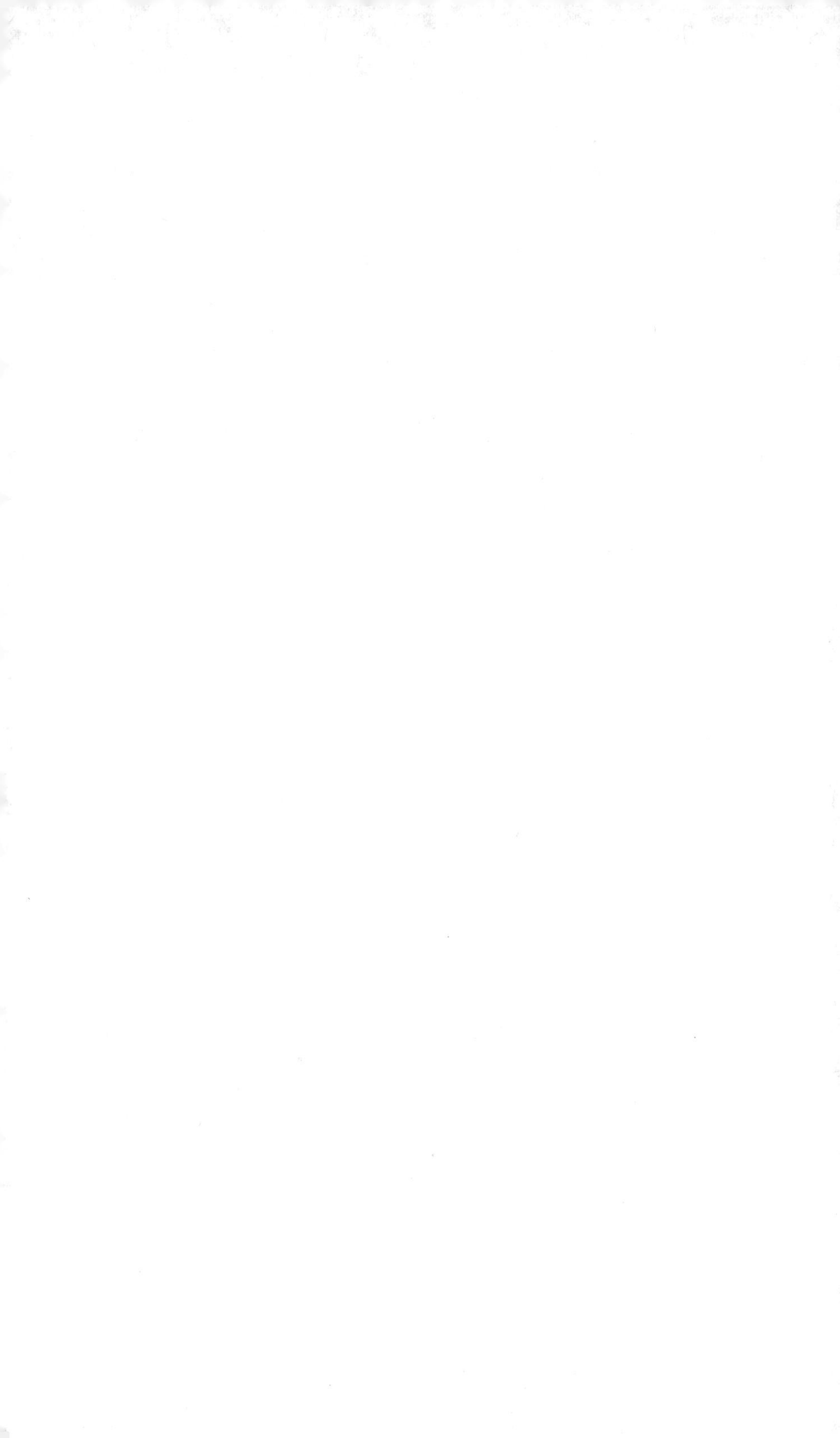

www.ingramcontent.com/pod-product-compliance
Lightning Source LLC
Chambersburg PA
CBHW071101260726
48661CB00006B/2395